Powerful Organic Ayurvedic Herbs to Strengthen Immunity

I0446565

Natural Ayurvedic Home

Remedies to Kill Viruses and

Boost Weak Immune System

Dan Phillips PhD

~DEDICATION~

~LARRY~

For your unwavering support, encouragement, and friendship. Your presence in my life has been a constant source of inspiration. Thank you for your invaluable kindness and belief in my journey. This book is a token of appreciation for your enduring friendship and steadfast encouragement.

TABLE OF CONTENT

CHAPTER 1. INTRODUCTION TO AYURVEDA AND IMMUNITY

  - EXPLORING THE FOUNDATIONAL PRINCIPLES OF AYURVEDA AND ITS EMPHASIS ON IMMUNITY.

  - UNDERSTANDING THE HOLISTIC APPROACH OF AYURVEDA TO MAINTAINING A STRONG IMMUNE SYSTEM.

CHAPTER 2. AYURVEDIC CONCEPT OF IMMUNITY AND HEALTH

  - DELVING INTO THE AYURVEDIC PERSPECTIVE ON IMMUNITY AND ITS CONNECTION TO OVERALL HEALTH.

  - DISCUSSING THE THREE DOSHAS (VATA, PITTA, KAPHA) AND THEIR ROLES IN IMMUNE FUNCTION.

CHAPTER 3. HERBS FOR IMMUNE SYSTEM ENHANCEMENT

- Highlighting specific organic Ayurvedic herbs renowned for boosting immunity.

- Detailing the properties and benefits of herbs like Ashwagandha, Tulsi (Holy Basil), and Amalaki (Indian Gooseberry).

Chapter 4. Ayurvedic Lifestyle Practices for Immune Support

- Exploring daily routines and practices that align with Ayurvedic principles to strengthen the immune system.

- Covering topics like balanced nutrition, proper sleep, and stress management.

Chapter 5. Natural Antiviral Ayurvedic Remedies

- Introducing potent antiviral herbs used in Ayurveda to combat viral infections.

- Providing guidance on using herbs like Neem, Turmeric, and Giloy for viral defense.

Chapter 6. Herbal Formulations and Recipes

- Offering Ayurvedic formulations and recipes that combine immune-boosting herbs for maximum efficacy.
- Sharing preparation methods for teas, tonics, and herbal blends.

Chapter 7. Seasonal Immunity Boosting Practices

- Discussing how Ayurveda adapts immunity enhancement strategies based on different seasons.
- Providing insights into seasonal changes and their impact on immune health.

Chapter 8. Integrating Ayurveda with Modern Wellness

- Exploring the integration of Ayurvedic practices with contemporary health approaches.
- Discussing ways to combine Ayurveda with exercise, meditation, and other wellness practices.

CHAPTER 1

Introduction to Ayurveda and Immunity

In a world when cutting-edge technology and modern medicine rule the day, people who seek balance and holistic well-being are nevertheless drawn to the age-old wisdom of Ayurveda. A deep understanding of the human body, mind, and spirit, as well as its complex relationship with the environment, is the foundation of Ayurveda. The core principle of

Ayurveda is the deep-rooted emphasis on immunity as the basis for overall well-being. This chapter introduces you to Ayurveda, revealing its guiding principles and shedding light on its all-encompassing method of building a strong immune system.

The Science of Life: Ayurveda

Known as the "Science of Life," Ayurveda is a traditional medical practice that has its roots in the Indian subcontinent and dates back thousands of years. An explanation of the name "Ayurveda" is found in Sanskrit, where "Ayur" means life and "Veda" means knowledge or science.

Ayurveda is essentially a holistic philosophy that takes into account one's mental, bodily, and spiritual health. It acknowledges that a condition of harmony and balance between the body, mind, and spirit is what true health is, rather than only the absence of disease.

Dosha System: Equilibrium of Elements

The Vata, Pitta, and Kapha doshas are three fundamental concepts in Ayurveda medicine that are used to explain immunity and health. The dynamic interaction of the five elements—earth, fire, water, and ether—is represented by these doshas. According to this belief, each person has an individual constitution, or "Prakriti," which is established by the relative strength of these doshas at the moment of birth. Restoring the equilibrium of these doshas is essential for good health and a robust immune system.

Ayurvedic Immunity: A Comprehensive View

Ayurveda takes a holistic approach to immunity, in contrast to the reductionist methods sometimes used in Western medicine. Immune system function is not limited to the physical body; it also includes the body's mental and spiritual integration. Ayurvedic literature highlights that healthy digestion, metabolism, and excretion are just a few of the body systems that work in unison to produce a robust immune system.

Ayurveda acknowledges that environmental factors, emotions, lifestyle choices, and dietary habits all have an impact on immunity. It recognizes the complex relationship between outside circumstances and internal health. Therefore, a person's immunity and general health are greatly influenced by their decisions and actions.

Ayurvedic Immunity Building

Ayurveda provides a thorough framework for strengthening and preserving a healthy immune system. This method goes beyond treating symptoms; instead, it seeks to identify the underlying causes of imbalances and makes customized interventions to resolve them.

Ayurveda's principal method of strengthening immunity is coordinating daily activities with the natural cycles of the day, or "dinacharya." This involves routines like waking up with the sun, taking care of oneself, and eating healthful meals at the right times. People can enhance the effective operation of their body systems and strengthen their immune systems by aligning with the cycles of nature.

Ayurveda also suggests attentive eating, which considers the properties of various foods as well as a person's constitution. Some foods, herbs, and spices, such amalaki (Indian gooseberry), ashwagandha, and tulsi (holy basil), are thought to have natural immune-boosting qualities.

Conclusion

With its holistic approach to immunological health that takes into account the body, mind, and spirit, Ayurveda is a shining example of ancient wisdom in a world where health issues are ever-present and changeable. It has the capacity to revolutionize our understanding of immunity because of its emphasis on balance, customized care, and alignment with natural rhythms.

It is crucial to understand the fundamental ideas of Ayurveda and its holistic viewpoint before we go into this investigation of potent organic Ayurvedic herbs to boost immunity. By exploring this ageless science, we give ourselves the means to develop a strong immune system and set out on a path to increased health and vigor.

CHAPTER 2

Ayurvedic Concept of Immunity and Health

The concept of immunity is woven into the very fabric of well-being in the complex tapestry of Ayurveda. Instead of being a stand-alone defense mechanism, immunity is the result of a dynamic interaction between several facets of the human physiology. The profound Ayurvedic understanding of immunity and its unbreakable link to general health is explored in this chapter. We examine how the three doshas—Pitta, Kapha, and Vata—affect immunological response and contribute to the overall balance that Ayurveda defines as wellbeing.

Immunity: The Keeper of Health

According to Ayurveda, immunity includes the mind and spirit in addition to the physical body's protection against outside invaders. When the internal ecology of a person is in a state of harmonious equilibrium, true immunity develops.

This includes having a calm mind, balanced doshas, optimal evacuation, and digestive fire (Agni). The body's vitality, resilience, and capacity to adjust to both internal and external changes are closely linked to immunity.

The Immune System and the Three Doshas

The three doshas—Vata, Pitta, and Kapha—are dynamic energies that regulate all physiological and psychological processes. They are the basis of Ayurveda's holistic approach to health. In the immune system, every dosha plays a unique function that together provide a cohesive protection against imbalances.

Immunity and Vata: The Protective Wind

Vata is the element of mobility and transformation and is ruled by the elements ether and air. It is the energy that makes intercellular communication possible, which is an essential component of immunological responses. Vata, when in balance, makes ensuring that immune cells are coordinated and immunological messages are delivered on time. On the other hand, an unbalanced Vata might result in unpredictable immunological reactions, which show themselves as hypersensitivity or a compromised defense.

Immunity and Pitta: The Flame of Change

Pitta represents metabolism and transformation and is associated with the elements of fire and water. It controls nutrition absorption, metabolism, and digestion—all processes that help the body become more resilient and immune. Toxins are efficiently removed from the body and immune cells are given the best possible nutrition when the Pitta is in balance. Conversely, an inflamed Pitta might result in immunological impairment and inflammation.

The Planet of Nourishment: Kappa and Immunity

As the sign of the earth and water elements, kapha represents stability and order. It gives the body protection, strength, and endurance. Kapha's capacity to erect a physical defense against infections is what gives it its role in immunity. Maintaining mucous membranes and other barriers of defense requires a balanced Kapha. Excess mucus production due to an unbalanced Kapha can cause congestion and increase the risk of respiratory infections.

Dosha Disproportion and Immune Function

Imbalances in any of the doshas might cause the immune system's delicate equilibrium to be upset. The method of treating immunity in Ayurveda focuses on balancing doshic constitution via individualised treatments. For example, grounding exercises, warm, nutritious foods, and peaceful hobbies help bring balance back to Vata imbalances. Cooling herbs and a well-balanced diet can help reduce inflammation and bring the immune system back into balance when Pitta is out of control. Breathing tonics, lightening foods, and energizing routines can all help restore energy to an imbalanced Kapha.

Finitude

The immune system is not a standalone entity but rather a complex dance of energies throughout the body, as the Ayurvedic concept of immunity reveals. The essential energies of Vata, Pitta, and Kapha are represented by the doshas, which have distinct but interrelated roles in this symphony of vitality and defense.

We discover as we go deeper into Ayurveda's knowledge that immunity is more than only protecting against outside dangers. When the mind is calm, Agni (digestive fire) is strong, and the doshas are in harmony, true immunity blossoms. The subtle beauty of Ayurveda's approach to health is demonstrated by this holistic viewpoint, which serves as a reminder that well-being is an orchestration of harmony, resilience, and balance.

CHAPTER 3

Herbs for Immune System
Enhancement

The natural world provides a wealth
of solutions for achieving vibrant
health and well-being. Ayurvedic
herbs are particularly effective in
bolstering the immune system and
promoting general well-being. This
chapter explores the world of

Ayurvedic herbs, which are well known for their extraordinary capacity to strengthen immunity. We'll look at the characteristics, advantages, and customs around a few herbs, such as amalaki (Indian gooseberry), tulsi (holy basil), and ashwagandha.

Ashwagandha: The Immunity Elixir

Celebrated for its adaptogenic properties, ashwagandha (Withania somnifera) is considered a cornerstone of Ayurvedic treatment. Adaptogens are essential nutrients that support the immune system by assisting the body in adjusting to stimuli and preserving equilibrium. Respected for its capacity to regulate the body's stress response, this plant also serves as an indirect immune system booster.

Moreover, ashwagandha is thought to have immunomodulatory qualities that boost immune cell function and encourage a strong resistance against infections. Packed with antioxidants, it fights inflammation and oxidative stress, which can weaken the immune system. Ashwagandha is a herb of choice for people looking for all-around immunological support because it is a tonic for energy.

Holy Basil (Tulsi): The Natural Immunomodulator

In Ayurveda, Tulsi (Ocimum sanctum), also referred to as Holy Basil, is a highly esteemed emblem of health and purity. Its long-standing repute as an immunomodulator is ingrained in custom. Flavonoids and essential oils are among the many phytochemicals that give tulsi its unique phytochemical profile and immune-boosting effects.

Because of its adaptogenic properties, tulsi supports immunological homeostasis and aids the body in managing stress. The antibacterial and anti-inflammatory properties of this substance enhance the body's resistance against infections. Regular Tulsi use is thought to enhance respiratory health, which makes it especially pertinent during periods when immune function is critical.

Indian gooseberry, or amalaki: The Nectar of Longevity

Thanks to its revitalizing and immune-boosting properties, Amalaki (Emblica officinalis), commonly known as Indian Gooseberry or Amla, has a special position in Ayurveda medicine. This little sour fruit is well known for having a high vitamin C content, which is essential for healthy immune system activity. The vitamin C in amalaki serves as an antioxidant, scavenging free radicals and advancing the health of cells.

Beyond just being high in vitamin C, amalaki also includes bioactive substances that boost immune cell activity. Its adaptogenic qualities promote resiliency and vitality by lessening the damaging effects of stress on the immune system. Amalaki is a classic herb for bolstering the body's defenses and promoting general health.

Unlocking the Potential: Combinations and Formulations that Work Together

When combined in harmonious mixtures and formulations, the power of Ayurvedic herbs is amplified. Ayurveda understands the potency of carefully mixing herbs to enhance their benefits. These combinations can address many facets of immune function in the context of immunity, guaranteeing a thorough approach.

A combination of amalaki, tulsi, and ashwagandha, for example, may have a symphony of immune-boosting benefits. The immune-modulatory qualities of Tulsi and Ashwagandha work in tandem, while the vitamin C in Amalaki enhances their effects by promoting cellular integrity. Combinations like this highlight Ayurveda's multifaceted approach to immunity.

Finitude

We discover a tapestry of time-tested natural medicines as we explore the world of Ayurvedic herbs for immune system development. Amalaki, Tulsi, and Ashwagandha stand out as three magnificent instances of gifts from nature that each bring something special to the immune system's harmonious composition.

These herbs have a major impact on immune system strength, balance, and resistance within the complex dance of the body's defense processes. Their historical applications, supported by current scientific knowledge, highlight their applicability to our pursuit of ideal health. We can develop a strong immune system that aids in our quest for vitality and well-being when we accept the wisdom of Ayurveda and its herbal companions.

CHAPTER 4

Ayurvedic Lifestyle Practices for Immune Support

- Exploring daily routines and practices that align with Ayurvedic principles to strengthen the immune system.

- Covering topics like balanced nutrition, proper sleep, and stress management.

Ayurveda invites us to embrace routines and attentive practices that create a tapestry of well-being in the rhythmic dance of life. This chapter provides a roadmap that takes us through the maze of Ayurvedic lifestyle practices that are specifically crafted to strengthen the immune system. Along the way, we will learn how to manage stress, embrace healthy sleep, and cultivate a balanced diet as we take a revolutionary step toward comprehensive immune support.

The Craft of Harmonious Eating

Ayurveda views nutrition as a celebration of nourishment that balances the body, mind, and soul rather than just providing for basic needs. Accept the wisdom of selecting foods based on what your body needs, the season, and your dosha are. Celebrate the range of nutrients found in fresh, healthy foods by consuming a rainbow of hues. Awareness of the six tastes—sweet, sour, salty, bitter, pungent, and astringent—must be developed because they provide a harmonious balance of nutrients and boost the immune system.

The Haven of Sound Sleep

Sleep is a precious place where the body and mind heal and regenerate, a sanctuary for regeneration. Ayurveda acknowledges the significant impact of sleep on immunological function. Make sleep a ritual, going to bed and waking up in sync with the cycles of the sun. Establish a peaceful bedtime routine that includes mindfulness exercises, relaxing herbal beverages, and gentle hobbies. Your immune system can flourish when you create a calm sleeping environment and respect your body's need for sleep.

Stress Reduction: The Balance Dance

Stress in today's hectic world might have a negative impact on immunological function. Ayurveda offers a variety of stress-reduction techniques that help patients regain their equilibrium. Learn the technique of breath control, or pranayama, to improve oxygenation and calm the nervous system. Practice mindfulness meditation and establish a sense of present-moment awareness. Think about using natural adaptogens, such as brahmi and ashwagandha, to strengthen your resistance to stress. You can cultivate an atmosphere that supports strong immune responses by learning to manage stress.

Daily Schedules: Creating Rhythms of Health and Well-Being

Dinacharya, the daily regimen prescribed by Ayurveda, acts as a guide for promoting health and harmony. Toxin removal and improved digestion can be achieved by starting your day with cleansing techniques like oil pulling and tongue scraping. Use dosha-balancing nourishing oils for self-massage (Abhyanga). Select activities that suit your constitution: vigorous exercises for Kapha, relaxing techniques for Pitta, and brisk walks for Vata. Set up regular meal times to improve absorption and digestion, and as the day comes to an end, relax with peaceful routines.

Developing Intentional Mindfulness

The practice of mindfulness, or being totally present, enhances all aspects of immune support. Eat with awareness, enjoying every taste and developing a relationship with the food you're consuming. Incorporate mindfulness into your everyday routine by appreciating the sound of falling leaves in the wind, the feel of warm water on your feet when you take a shower, and other small sensory experiences. Through the practice of mindful awareness, you can develop immunological resilience by developing a closer relationship with your body's signals and demands.

Finitude

We discover the secrets to building a strong immune system in the haven of Ayurvedic lifestyle practices. The cornerstones of wellbeing are stress management, regular routines, mindfulness, balanced eating, and sound sleep. We respect the complex dance that our bodies, thoughts, and spirits perform, as well as how they are connected to the rhythms of the natural world, as we walk this road.

These activities are not isolated ones; rather, they are the threads that weave a vibrant and harmonic symphony. When we accept Ayurveda's invitation to live according to its ageless precepts, we step into a world where everything we do is a note in the vast orchestration of immune support that is holistic. We set out on a life-changing journey towards enduring well-being through the art of Ayurvedic living, where the bright glow of health is cultivated from within.

CHAPTER 5

Natural Antiviral Ayurvedic Remedies

- Introducing potent antiviral herbs used in Ayurveda to combat viral infections.

- Providing guidance on using herbs like Neem, Turmeric, and Giloy for viral defense.

Facing viral assaults that persistently jeopardize human health, Ayurvedic wisdom provides a wealth of natural antiviral treatments. This section explores the world of powerful Ayurvedic herbs that act as watchful guardians against viral infections. In addition to offering priceless advice on maximizing the potency of important antiviral herbs like giloy, neem, and turmeric for strong virus defense, we will examine the characteristics, advantages, and traditional applications of these plants.

Neem: The Viral Shield of Nature

Neem (Azadirachta indica) is a powerful antiviral weapon in the Ayurvedic toolbox. Neem, revered for ages for its antimicrobial properties and bitter taste, has been used to fight illnesses. It is a flexible ally in the battle against viral invaders because of its broad range of antiviral characteristics.

Neem's antiviral properties are attributed to its components, including nimbin and nimbidin, which disrupt the process of viral reproduction. Furthermore, neem helps the body develop a strong defense by bolstering the immune system's reaction to infections. Adding Neem to everyday routines—whether by local application, oral ingestion, or even neem-infused oils—can strengthen the body's defenses against viruses.

Golden Shield of Turmeric Against Viruses

In Ayurveda, turmeric (Curcuma longa), renowned for both its healing qualities and vivid golden hue, is another reliable antiviral herb. Turmeric's main ingredient, curcumin, has drawn notice for its wide range of antiviral properties. It stops viruses from replicating and from entering host cells, hence halting the spread of diseases.

The immune-modulating properties of turmeric amplify its antiviral efficacy. Turmeric helps the body identify and get rid of viral threats more efficiently by enhancing immunological responses. Adding turmeric to regular meals, teas, or golden milk elixirs strengthens the body's defenses against viruses and promotes general health.

The Immune-Boosting Elixir: Giloy

Tinospora cordifolia, or giloy, is a highly prized herb in Ayurveda, valued for its antiviral and immune-stimulating properties. Giloy, often called "Amrita" or the "root of immortality," has long been utilized to strengthen immunity to disease. It boosts the immune system's development and function, strengthening the body's defenses.

The capacity of goloy to prevent viral attachment and penetration into host cells is thought to be the source of its antiviral qualities. Giloy slows the spread of diseases by stopping the viral life cycle. When taken as powders, capsules, or decoctions, Giloy provides a strong defense against viral invaders and enhances health and energy.

Unlocking the Antiviral Potential: Real-World Uses

Strengthening viral defense can be achieved in a concrete way by incorporating these antiviral herbs into everyday practices. Using neem, turmeric, and giloy to their full potential requires innovative uses that optimize their health advantages.

Neem: To encourage antiviral activity, use neem leaves, neem oil, or neem supplements. Neem-infused creams and lotions provide topical protection, while mouthwashes and oils with neem as an ingredient promote dental health.

Curry powder: Golden milk, drinks, and foods infused with turmeric spice will elevate your culinary adventures. Turmeric tablets offer concentrated advantages, while oils and cosmetics items packed with turmeric offer external support.

Giloy: Take use of giloy's ability to strengthen immunity by using tinctures, pills, or powders. Make nutritious tonics using giloy or add it to other herbs for a synergistic effect.

Finitude

Ayurveda offers a wealth of information in the field of natural antiviral therapies that is timeless and gives hope to those facing viral difficulties. Strong protectors like neem, turmeric, and giloy each have special qualities that strengthen the body's defenses against viral invaders.

Discovering a wealth of health-promoting customs, we go through the Ayurvedic antiviral herb tapestry. By incorporating these herbs into our daily routine, we can strengthen our immunity and develop a strong bond with the restorative force of nature. We give ourselves the ability to move across the complex terrain of viral dangers with resiliency, strength, and a fresh lease on life by embracing these natural partners.

CHAPTER 6

Herbal Formulations and Recipes

- Offering Ayurvedic formulations and recipes that combine immune-boosting herbs for maximum efficacy.

- Sharing preparation methods for teas, tonics, and herbal blends.

Starting a journey of immune-boosting Ayurvedic medicines opens the door to a whole new realm of well-being. This chapter explores the technique of creating herbal recipes and formulations that combine immune-boosting herbs in a way that maximizes their potency. For the best possible immune support, we investigate the alchemical fusion of nature's treasures through nourishing teas, energizing tonics, and harmonious herbal blends.

The Boosting Effects of Herbal Combinations on Immunity

Ayurveda's wisdom is typified by its precise proportionate use of plant combinations. Herbs when combined harmoniously provide a symphony that enhances each one of their unique benefits. Consider mixing herbs such as amalaki, tulsi, and ashwagandha to boost immunity. Tulsi's immunomodulatory properties are enhanced by ashwagandha's adaptogenic qualities, while Amalaki's vitamin C content increases cellular integrity. Create a blend that is in harmony with your needs and constitution.

Energizing Immune Tonics: A Resilience Recipe

You can use an immune-stimulating tonic as a daily immune-supporting drink. Mix equal portions of Giloy, Shatavari (Asparagus racemosus), and ashwagandha. Shatavari promotes energy, ashwagandha builds resistance, and giloy strengthens the immune system. For all-around immune support, steep these herbs in water, filter, and drink this tonic every day. Honey can be added to sweeten for a tasty variation.

Teas for Boosting Immunity: Vitality Infusions

Drinking herbal teas is a calming custom that is good for the body and the spirit. Make a revitalizing immune tea with licorice (Glycyrrhiza glabra), turmeric, and neem. Turmeric modulates the immune system, neem offers antiviral protection, and licorice improves the synergy of herbs. Add these herbs to a cup of hot water, steep, and drink with awareness. Add some ginger or lemon for extra taste and health benefits.

External and Internal Immunity with Radiant Skin Elixir

The largest organ in the body, the skin, is essential to immunity. Create a remedy that supports health from the inside out. Mix the gel of Aloe Vera (Aloe barbadensis), Turmeric, and Neem. Aloe Vera calms, turmeric encourages healthy skin, and neem's antiviral qualities shield. For glowing skin and inner vitality, take this mixture internally and apply topically.

Herbal Ghee: A Powerful Shot of Nutrients

In Ayurveda, clarified butter, or ghee, is a highly esteemed carrier of herbal properties. Infuse clarified butter with Brahmi (Bacopa monnieri), turmeric, and ashwagandha to make a powerful herbal ghee. Brahmi improves mental health, turmeric supports the immune system, and ashwagandha increases energy. Use this herbal ghee in your cooking or just take a tablespoon every day to support your body and mind.

Heating Immune Elixir: Balancing Kapha

In seasons when Kapha is predominant, a warming immune elixir might offer essential equilibrium. Blend cardamom, ginger, and cinnamon together for an energizing combination. Cardamom adds depth to aroma, cinnamon encourages circulation, and ginger lights the fire in the digestive system. These spices should be steamed in water, strained, and then honey-sweetened. Drink this elixir to boost immunity and counteract the dampening effects of Kapha.

Finitude

Within the framework of Ayurvedic medicine, the skill of creating herbal formulas and recipes takes on a creative and nurturing role. Through the synergistic blending of immune-boosting herbs, we can fully unleash the medicinal power of nature's precious resources. Every product, from adaptable ghee infusions to calming teas and energizing tonics, reflects the goal of promoting complete well-being.

Upon accepting the habit of mixing herbs and incorporating them into regular routines, you set out on a path of self-realization and empowerment. These mixtures become more than just mixtures; they represent your collaboration with the wisdom of nature. By using the alchemical properties of herbs, you can strengthen your defenses against illness, develop energy, and become the embodiment of the balanced harmony that is the foundation of Ayurveda.

CHAPTER 7

Seasonal Immunity Boosting

Practices

- Discussing how Ayurveda adapts immunity enhancement strategies based on different seasons.

- Providing insights into seasonal changes and their impact on immune health.

The seasons work in unison to create a dance between the natural world and our physical selves that profoundly affects our overall health. With its profound linkages to the cycles of nature, Ayurveda understands that every season offers new possibilities for strengthening the immune system as well as special obstacles. This chapter delves into the ways in which Ayurveda modifies immunity-boosting techniques according to the seasons, providing valuable perspectives on the intricate relationship between immunological health and the cycles of nature.

The Changing Relationship: Immune Health and Seasons

Our bodies are microcosms of the greater macrocosm of the cosmos, as Ayurveda recognizes. We experience internal environment shifts in reaction to the changing of the seasons. The potency and adaptability of our immune system may be affected by these changes. We can enhance our immune system and general health by adjusting our habits and behaviors to the seasonal changes.

Fall and Early Winter are Vata Seasons

Vata season winds bring with them a tendency toward dryness and instability. The integrity of the immune system may be jeopardized by this. During this season, Ayurveda encourages grounding activities to counterbalance Vata's unpredictable tendency. Rich foods, warming spices, and regular self-massage with sesame oil provide immune system stability and support.

Sudden Winter and Early Spring: Kapha Season

As Kapha season approaches, moisture and congestion could pose a threat to the health of the immune system. Activities that promote circulation and balance Kapha are recommended by Ayurveda. Exercises that are vigorous, a lighter diet, and the use of warming spices like black pepper and ginger help counteract Kapha's tendency to stifle the immune system.

Summer is Pitta Season

The intense heat during Pitta season can lead to irritation and discomfort. During this period, cooling techniques are necessary for immune balance.

Staying hydrated, using cooling herbs like mint and coriander, and engaging in soothing activities all help to keep your immune system robust during the summer.

Switching Seasons: Adjusting with Intelligence

The seasons of spring and fall signal changes in the relative dominance of the doshas. The body experiences particular difficulties at these times as it adjusts to shifting energy. During these periods, detoxification techniques like Ayurvedic cleansing rituals (Panchakarma) aid in the immune system's reset and optimal performance.

Symphonizing with the Seasons: A Comprehensive Method

Seasonal practices in Ayurveda cover the mind and spirit in addition to diet and lifestyle modifications. Practicing seasonal attention, meditation, and pranayama (breath control) facilitates the synchronization of internal and external cycles. This balance strengthens immunological responses by creating a sense of resonance with nature.

Finitude

The seasons are chapters in the Ayurvedic tapestry that contain deep knowledge for strengthening immunity. Understanding how Vata, Kapha, and Pitta energies affect our bodies helps us to unlock the secrets of a healthy immune system. We dance with nature to establish optimal well-being by adjusting our routines, nutrition, and practices to match the changing seasons.

By embracing the seasonal immunity-boosting practices of Ayurveda, you set out on a path of cosmic attunement. You may respect the ancient knowledge and strengthen your immune system from the inside out by approaching each season with awareness and intention. This chapter extends an invitation to you to embrace the seasonal rhythms and discover the transforming power of synchronizing with nature's cycles for resilience and lifelong vitality.

CHAPTER 8

Integrating Ayurveda with Modern Wellness

- Exploring the integration of Ayurvedic practices with contemporary health approaches.

- Discussing ways to combine Ayurveda with exercise, meditation, and other wellness practices.

Through the harmonious fusion of traditional knowledge and cutting-edge research, a potent route to comprehensive well-being is revealed through the synthesis of Ayurveda and modern health methods. This chapter explores the art of integrating Ayurvedic principles with contemporary health practices in a seamless manner, providing information on how Ayurveda can complement wellness techniques such as meditation, exercise, and other activities for a well-rounded and balanced existence.

The Body, Mind, and Spirit Working Together

The fundamental principle of Ayurveda is the understanding of the interdependence of the body, mind, and spirit. The advantages of any undertaking are increased when this holistic viewpoint is combined with contemporary wellness techniques. Ayurveda adds depth and intention to wellness activities like exercise, meditation, and other interests, making people feel more unified and purposeful.

Workout: Harmonious Movement

Being physically active is essential to wellbeing. When exercise is aligned with Ayurvedic principles, it turns into a balancing art. The effectiveness of your fitness regimen is increased if it is in line with your dominant dosha or the current season. Grounding exercises like yoga and strolling are beneficial for Vata folks; cooling exercises like swimming are beneficial for Pitta individuals; and dynamic workouts like dance or vigorous climbing are beneficial for Kapha individuals.

Meditation: Developing Inner Calm

Finding inner peace can be accessed through meditation. Meditation is enhanced by Ayurveda, which customizes techniques based on personal constitutions and imbalances. Grounding meditation techniques can be comforting for Vata types; cooling visualization can be beneficial for Pitta types; and breathwork can be energizing for Kapha types. The customized method of Ayurveda enhances meditation and fosters emotional equilibrium and mental clarity.

Diet & Nutrition: A Blend of Innovation & Tradition

The emphasis on mindful eating in Ayurveda and modern nutrition go hand in hand. You may establish nutritious harmony in your meal planning by incorporating Ayurvedic concepts. When choosing foods, take into account your body's demands, the season, and your dosha. For best effects, try customizing common food fads, such as intermittent fasting, to fit your specific Ayurvedic profile.

Stress Reduction: The Way to Calm

Stress is a problem that affects everyone, and Ayurveda has a wealth of remedies for managing stress. The effectiveness of Ayurvedic relaxation techniques like self-massage

(Abhyanga) and oil application on the forehead (Shirodhara) is increased when incorporated into contemporary stress-reduction strategies. By balancing doshic imbalances, these activities provide a foundation of peace that makes one resilient to life's challenges.

Whole-Body Healing: A Path to Wholeness

The self-care rituals of Ayurveda are in harmony with contemporary practices, nourishing the complete person. A customised haven of wellbeing can be created by using herbal self-massage, scented baths, and daily activities that are catered to your dosha. You develop an inner sense of fullness that shines out when you include these techniques into your everyday routine.

Finitude

The fusion of Ayurveda and contemporary wellness signifies the dawn of a new age in holistic health. By combining information from today with the wisdom of the past, you create a route that is deep, balanced, and purposeful. You can take a transformative journey that respects tradition and embraces the dynamic nature of the present by incorporating Ayurvedic principles into your exercise, meditation, nutrition, stress management, and self-care routines.

Ayurveda becomes a golden thread that weaves harmony and vigor into every aspect of your life. The possibility of experiencing comprehensive well-being in its purest form—a bright symphony of mind, body, and spirit in perfect harmony—awakens as you combine Ayurveda with contemporary wellness.